If Men Had Babies...

by
Karen Rostoker-Gruber
and
Gail Panzer-Salmanowitz

illustrated by
Jim Gallagher

CCC Publications

Published by

CCC Publications
9725 Lurline Avenue
Chatsworth, CA 91311

Manufactured in the United States of America.

Cover © 2001 CCC Publications.

Interior illustrations © 2001 CCC Publications.

Cover & interior art by Jim Gallagher.

Cover & interior production by Continental Imaging Center.

ISBN 1-57644-123-7

If your local bookstore is out of stock, copies of this book may be obtained by mailing check or money order for $7.99 per book (plus $2.75 to cover postage and handling) to: CCC Publications, 9725 Lurline Avenue, Chatsworth, CA 91311.

Pre-publication Edition - 8/01

DEDICATIONS

A special thanks to Cliff Carle, without whose patience and humor
this book would not be what it is today.
❧

This book is dedicated to my husband, Scott; my daughter, Michelle;
my mother and father, Earl and Marge; my sister, Dawn; my cousins, Ronni and Tracie;
and my friends Andrea Ferreira, Claudia and Ann Porzio Lewis,
who always reads countless revisions of my work.

Karen Rostoker-Gruber
❧

To my husband, Dennis; my kids, Christina, Rebecca, Emily, Dennis and Jason;
my parents, Sandy and Alvin Panzer, and my brother, Michael.

Gail Panzer-Salmanowitz
❧

To my wife, Donna; my kids, Dylan and Jimmy, and my mother, Mary.

Jim Gallagher

INTRODUCTION

Have you ever wondered what life after baby would be like if women were the ones who got to watch TV, drink beer, eat beer nuts, and lounge around—and MEN had to do the grocery shopping, cook nutritious meals, put in loads of laundry, give baths, change diapers, and sing lullabies for hours on end? Find out how different life would be if the tables were turned and MEN HAD BABIES!!!

If Men Had Babies...

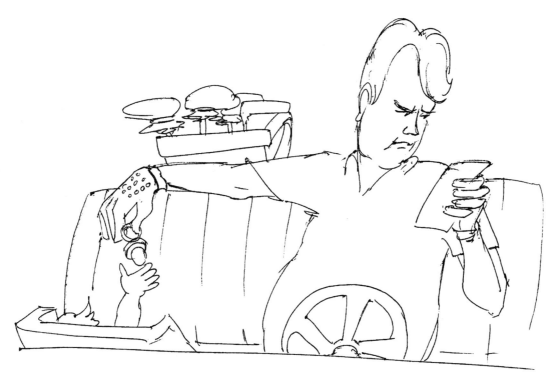

golf carts would come equipped with car seats.

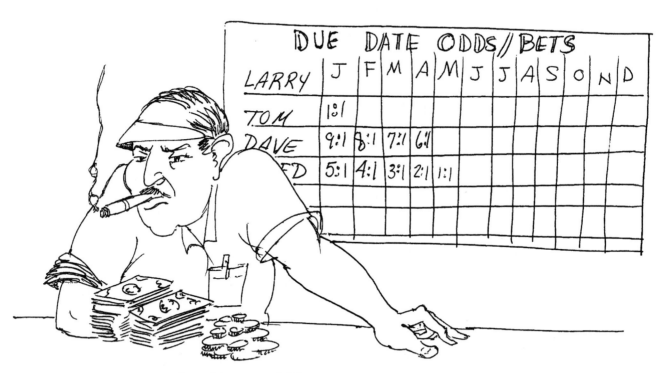

bookies would have a line on due dates.

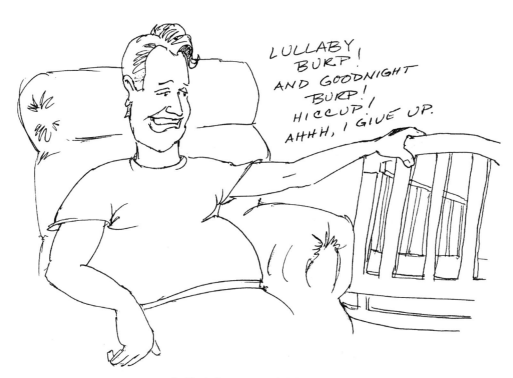

lullabies would be burped.

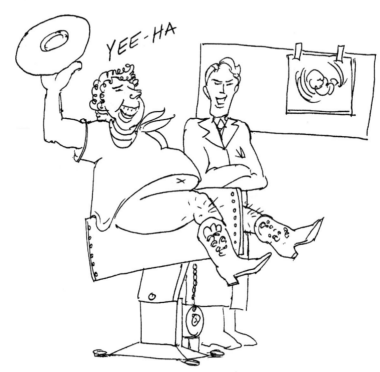

examination tables would operate like mechanical bucking bulls.

If Men Had Babies...

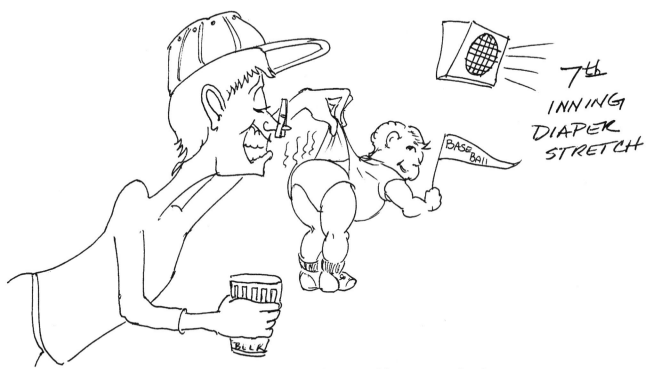

diapers would only get changed between innings.

If Men Had Babies...

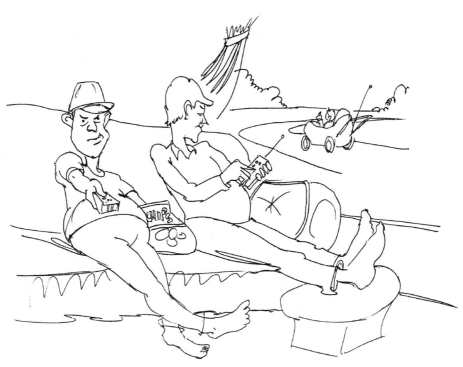

carriages would resemble remote-controlled mini sports cars.

If Men Had Babies...

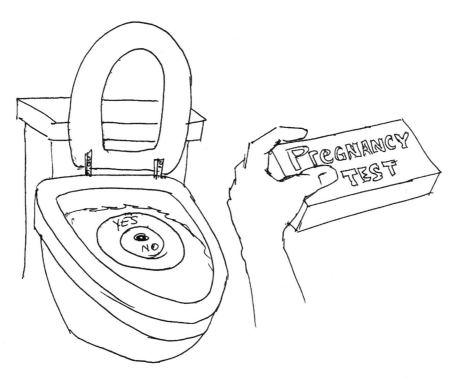

pregnancy tests would be flushable, floating toilet targets.

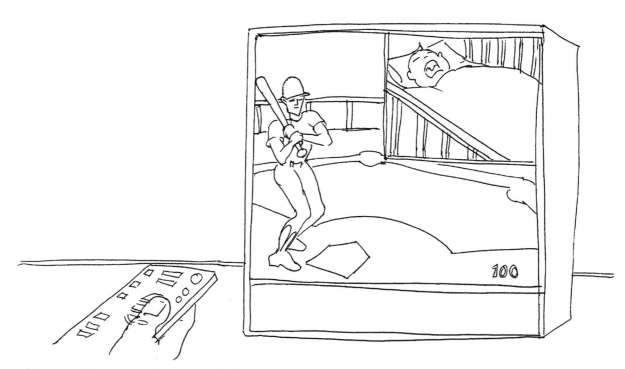

video baby monitors would have 150 channels and picture-in-picture screens.

If Men Had Babies...

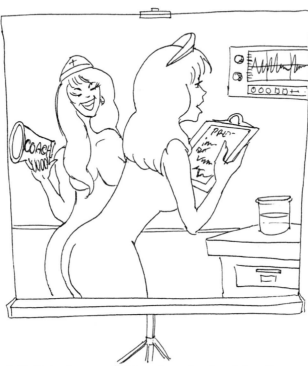

videos on natural childbirth would be loaded with plenty of naked nurses.

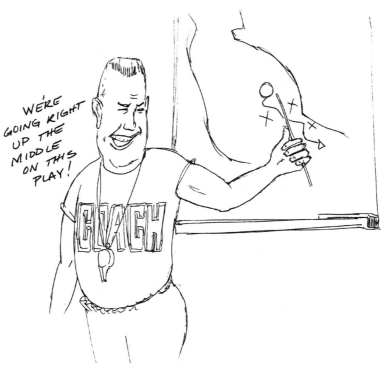

Lamaze would be taught play-by-play.

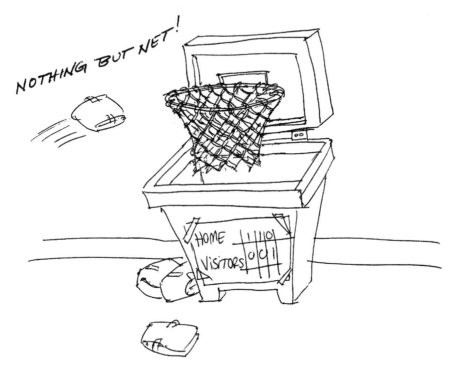

all diaper pails would come equipped with basketball hoops.

If Men Had Babies...

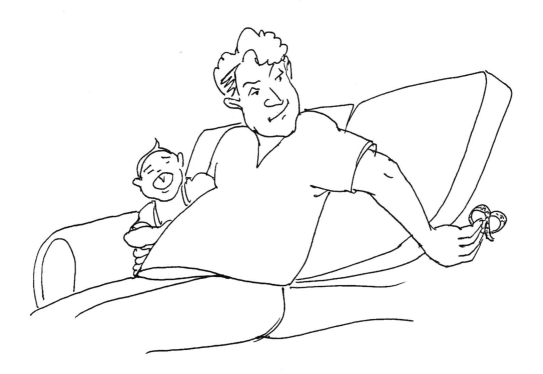

teething rings would actually be stale pretzels left over from the Super Bowl.

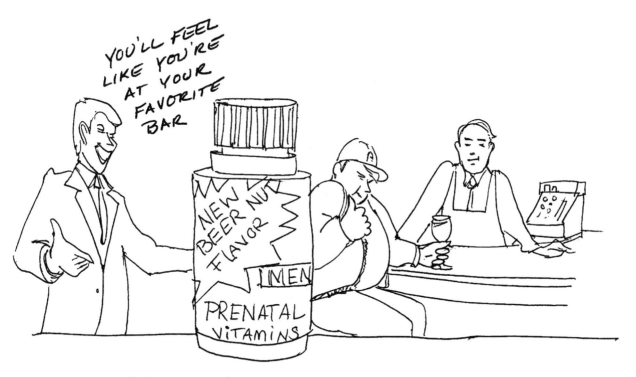

their prenatal vitamins would taste like beer nuts.

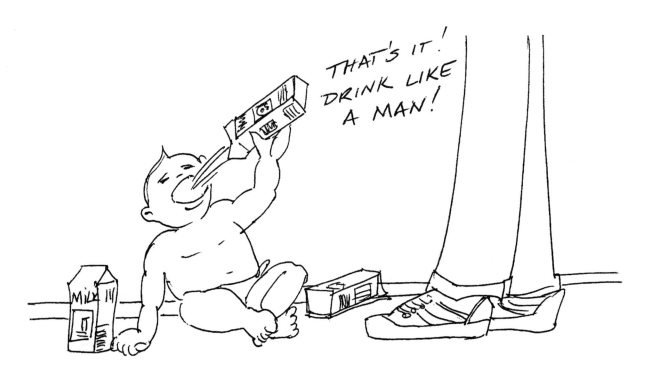

babies would have to learn to drink directly out of milk cartons.

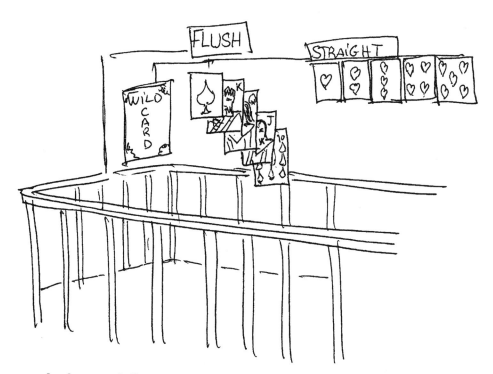

baby mobiles would teach kids how to count cards.

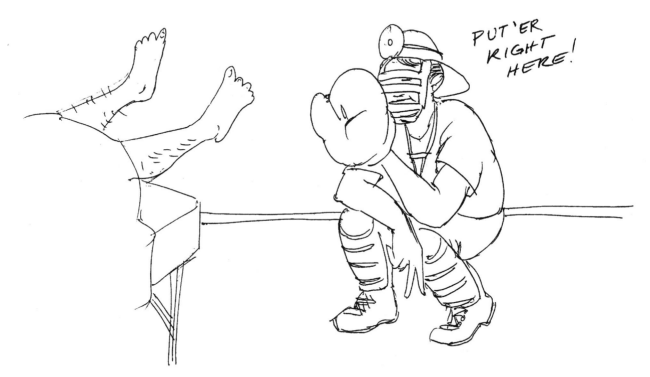

deliveries would be performed with catcher's mitts.

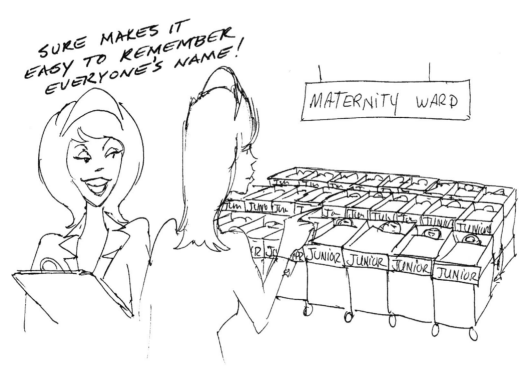

each and every baby would be named Junior.

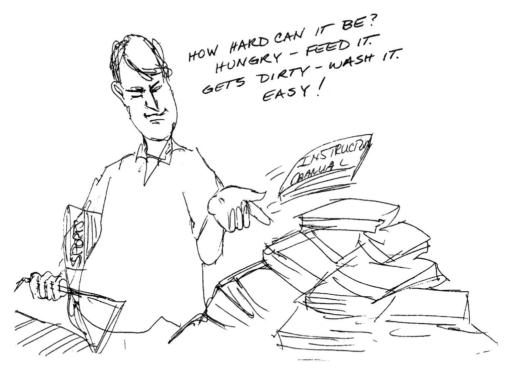

babies would come with instruction manuals — but no guy would read them.

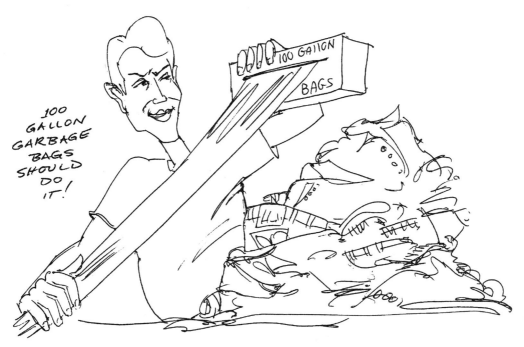

since washing machines don't operate by remote control,
all baby clothes would have to be disposable.

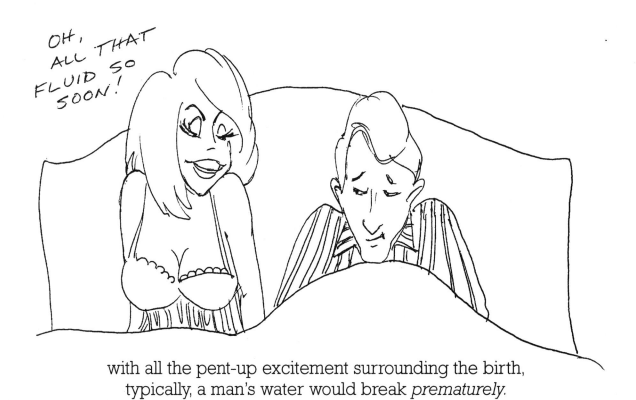

with all the pent-up excitement surrounding the birth,
typically, a man's water would break *prematurely*.

If Men Had Babies...

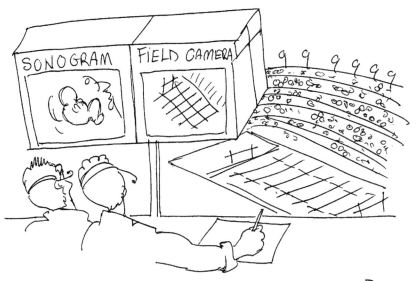

sonograms would have instant replay.

If Men Had Babies...

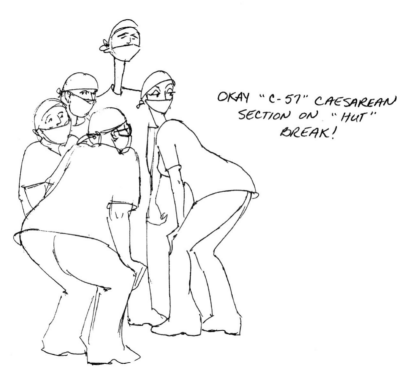

OKAY "C-57" CAESAREAN SECTION ON "HUT" BREAK!

before a delivery, doctors and nurses would get together in a huddle.

If Men Had Babies...

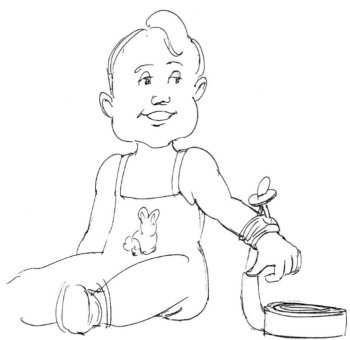

to save time searching for lost pacifiers,
men would just duct tape them to their babies' hands.

If Men Had Babies...

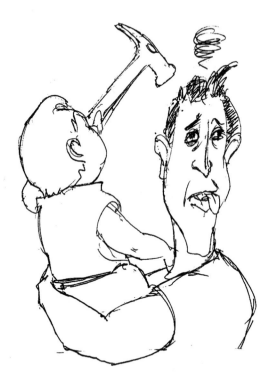

all rattles would be shaped like something manly. . . hammers, screwdrivers, or pliers.

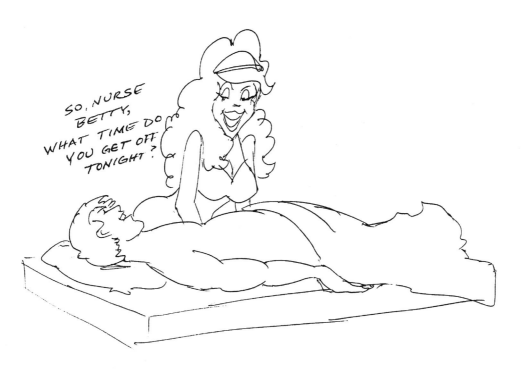

they would even flirt while getting a C-section.

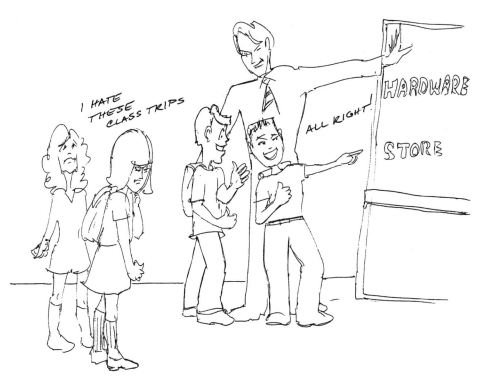

all class trips would be to the local hardware store.

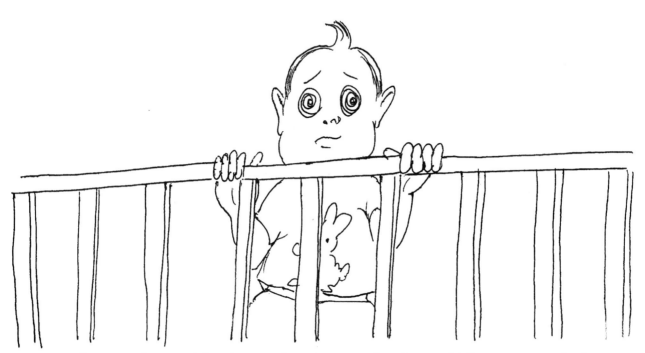

the two-hour videotapes that are used to keep kids preoccupied would be redesigned to run ten hours straight.

If Men Had Babies...

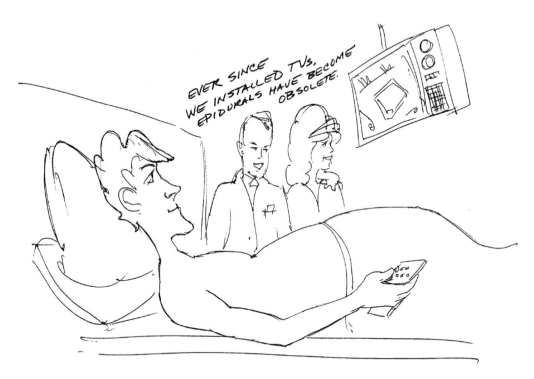

without exception, delivery rooms would have TVs mounted on the ceiling.

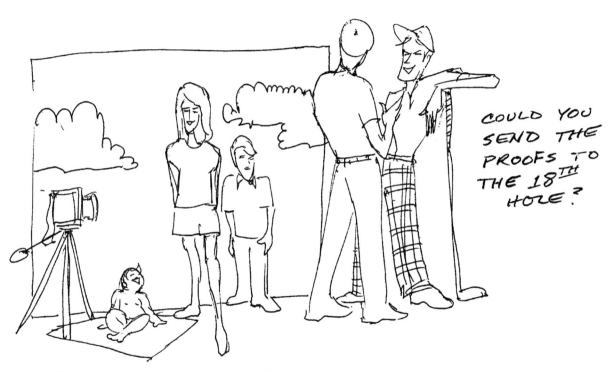

instead of portrait studios at the mall, they'd be located at the local golf course.

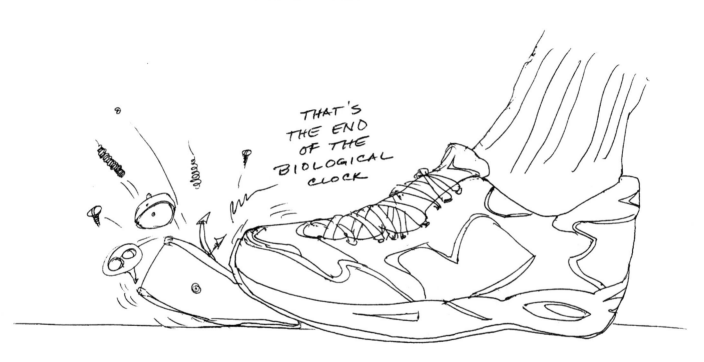

the concept of "biological clocks" would disappear—after all,
men have no concept of time.

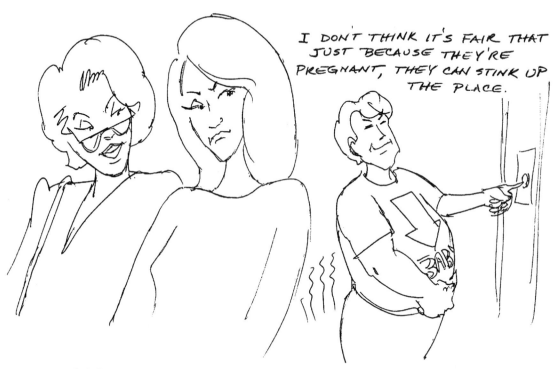

pregnancy would finally give men a valid excuse for burping and farting in public.

If Men Had Babies...

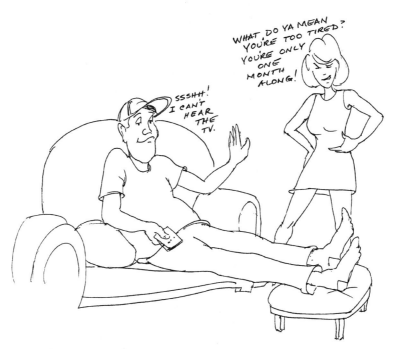

instead of bed rest in the eighth month,
mandatory "couch rest" would start immediately.

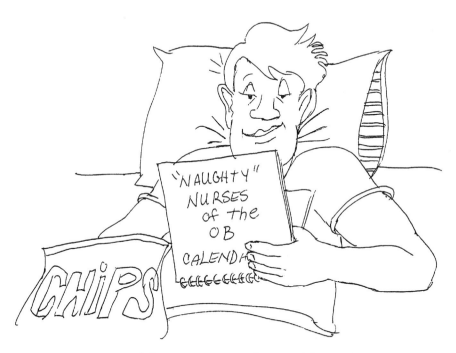

recovery rooms would come complete with recliners, beer, chips, big screen TVs, and naked pictures of the OB nursing staff.

If Men Had Babies...

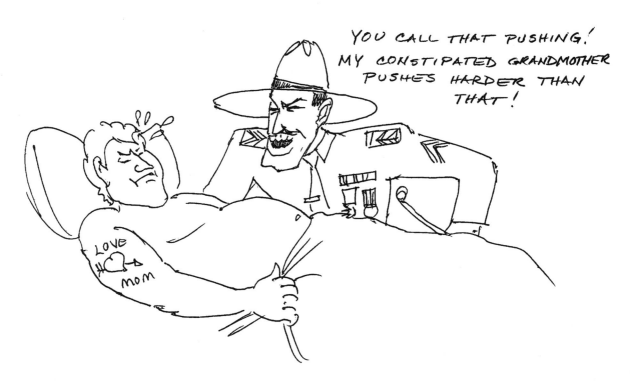

delivery coaches would be ex-marine drill sergeants.

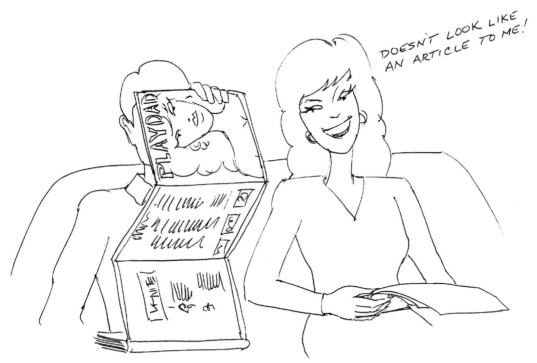

they would claim to buy "girly" magazines only for the pregnancy articles.

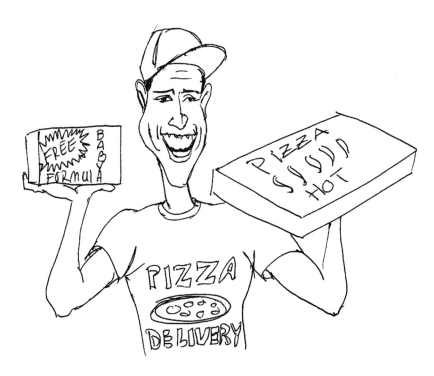

pizza parlors would offer "free formula" with every large pie.

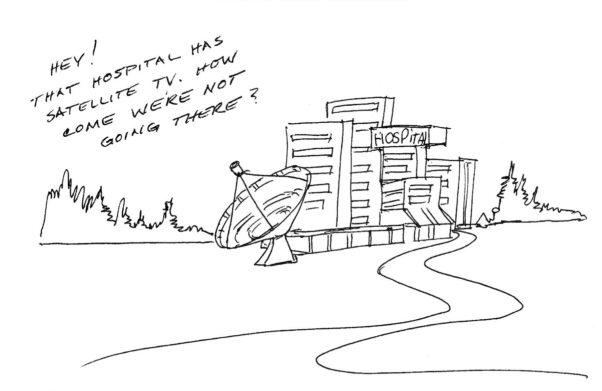

their first question at the hospital would be, "Do you have cable?"

If Men Had Babies...

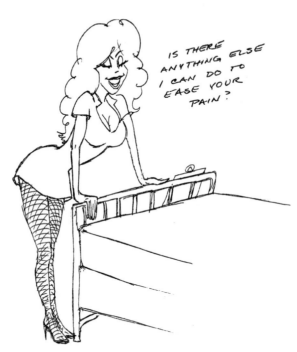

all OB nurses would be required to wear fishnet stockings, stiletto heels, and white miniskirts.

If Men Had Babies...

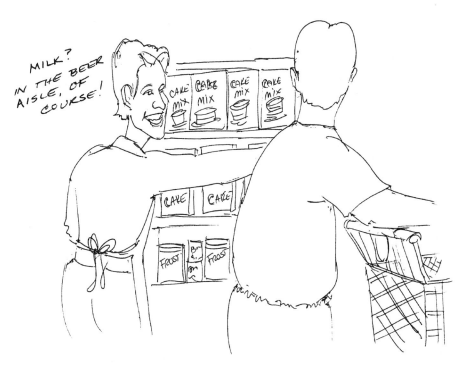

to remind them to pick it up, milk would be found only in the beer case.

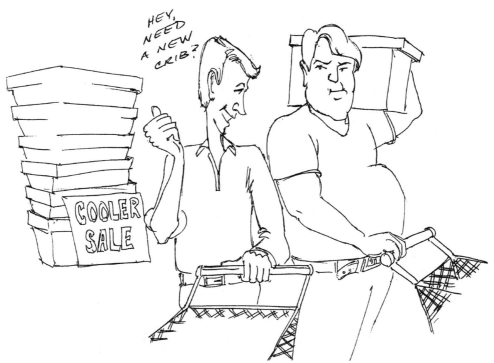

all baby carriers would resemble beer coolers.

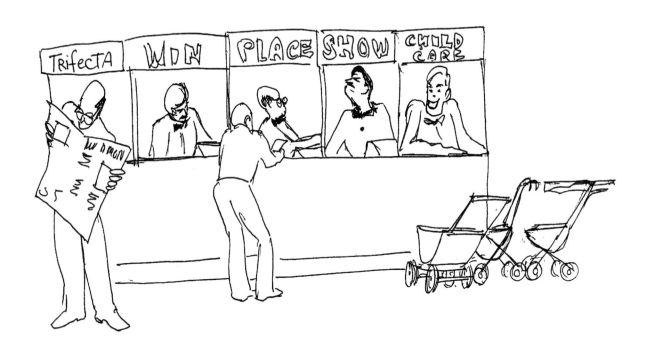

racetracks would have daycare centers.

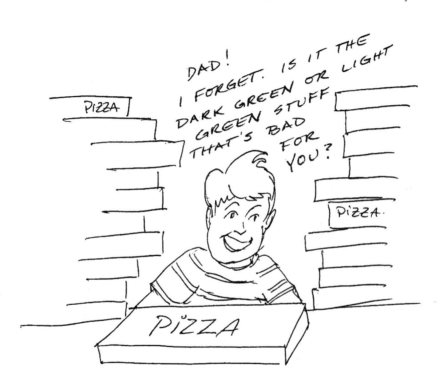

there'd be only one after-school snack: leftover pizza.

If Men Had Babies...

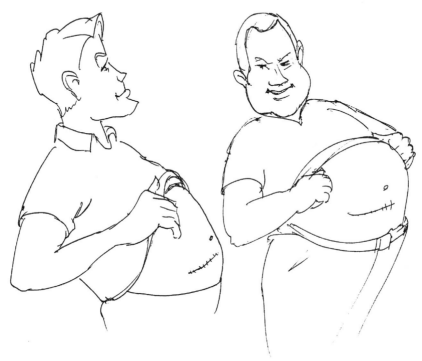

because size DOES MATTER, C-section scars would have to be longer than *six inches*.

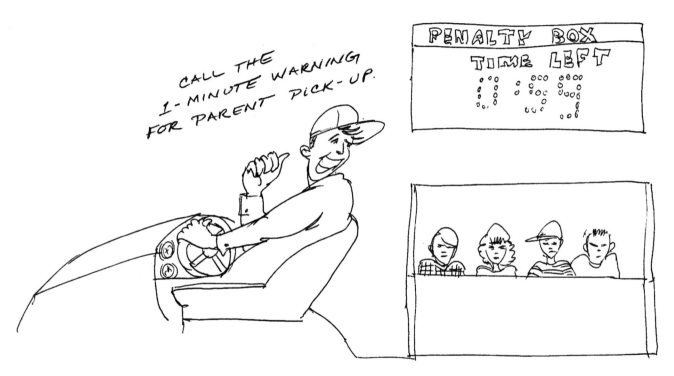

instead of a "time-out," kids would be sent to penalty boxes.

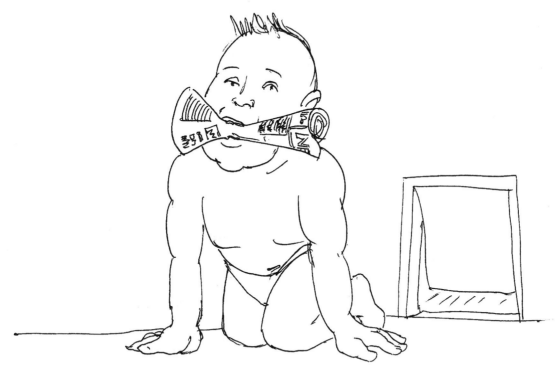

as soon as they could walk, babies would be trained to get the Sunday paper.

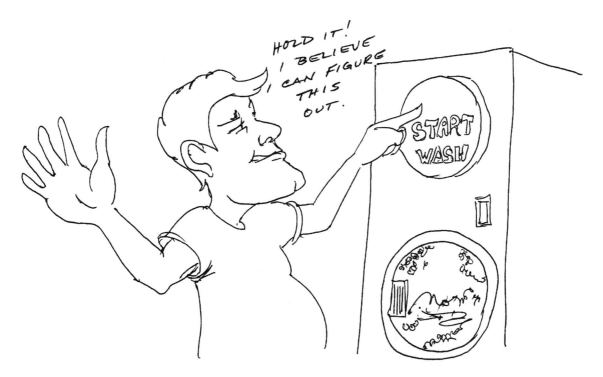

laundry machines would have only one button... "START."

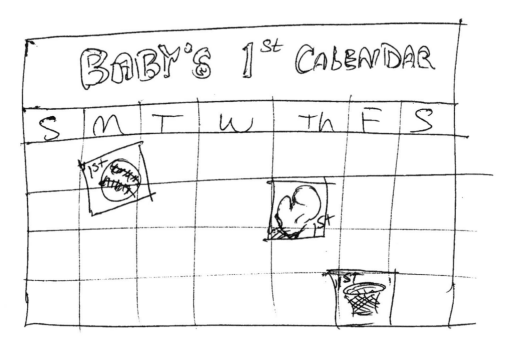

baby's first-year calendar would be drastically different:
first ball game, first fistfight, first mud-wrestling contest.

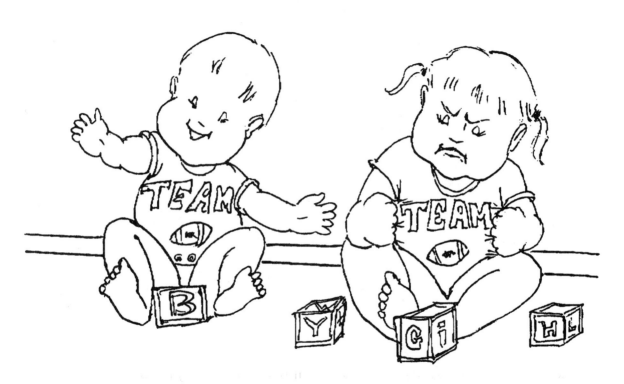

all baby clothes would come with team logos.

If Men Had Babies...

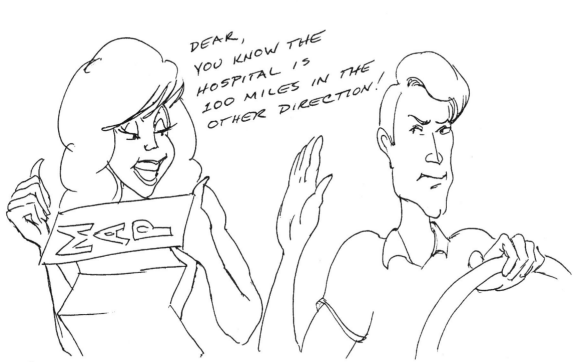

no matter how strong the contractions were, if they got lost on the way to the hospital, they'd still refuse to stop and ask for directions.

If Men Had Babies...

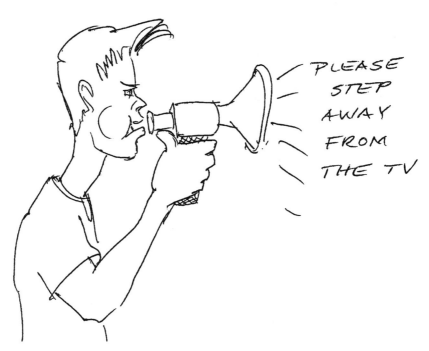

PLEASE STEP AWAY FROM THE TV

there would be no need for childproofing, since most men just own
a refrigerator, recliner, TV, and a toilet.

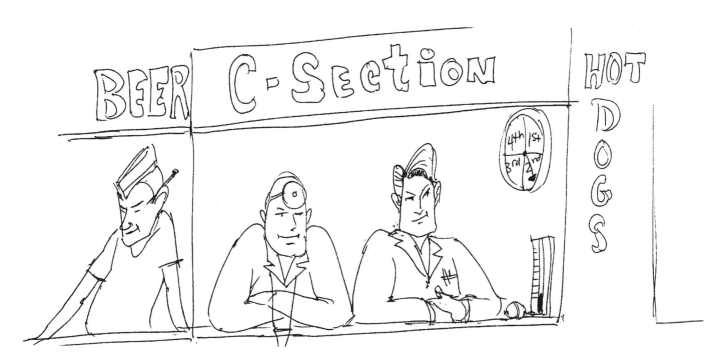

they would all demand C-sections so they could schedule their deliveries during halftime.

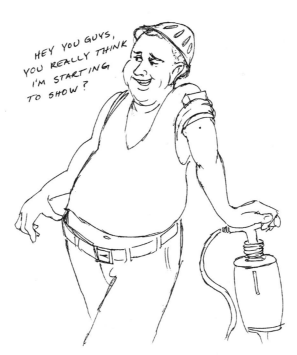

there'd be no need for maternity clothes.
Men would just keep pushing their belts down lower and lower.

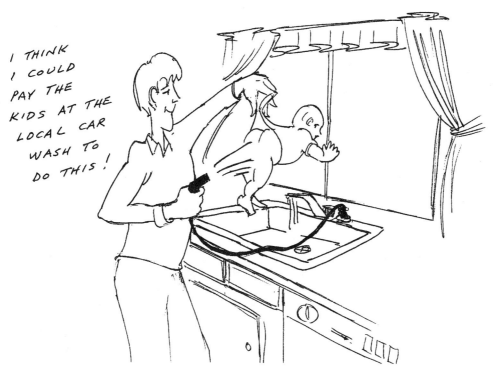

instead of giving babies baths, they'd just hose them down.

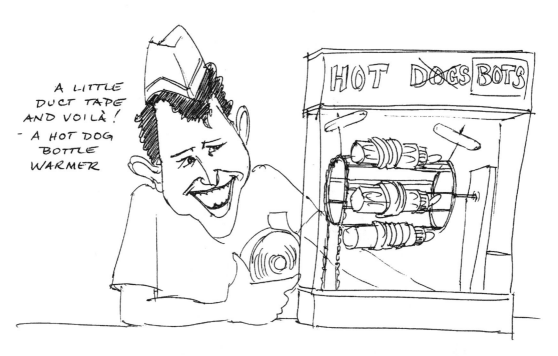

since fathers would have to bring their babies EVERYWHERE,
all concession stands would begin serving warm bottles of milk.

If Men Had Babies...

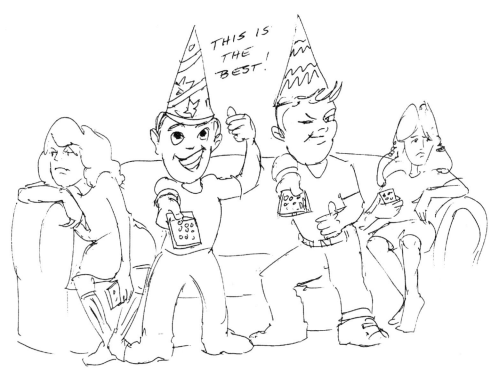

this is what a typical boy's birthday party would look like. . .

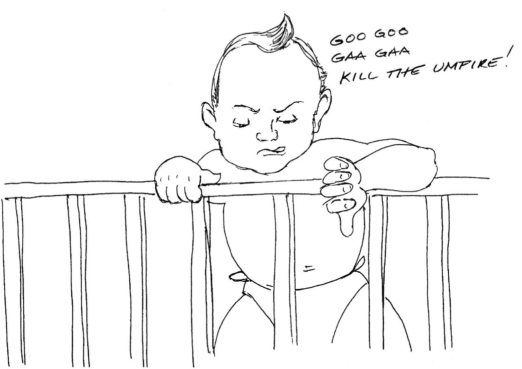

baby's first words would be: "Kill the umpire!"

If Men Had Babies...

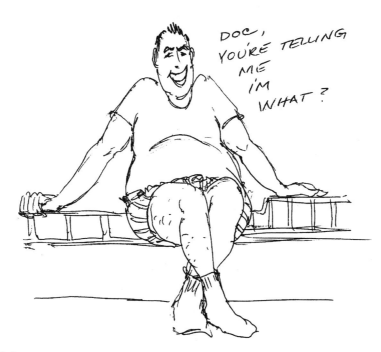

they wouldn't even know they were pregnant. As they gain weight, they'll figure it's from too many beer nuts and chips.

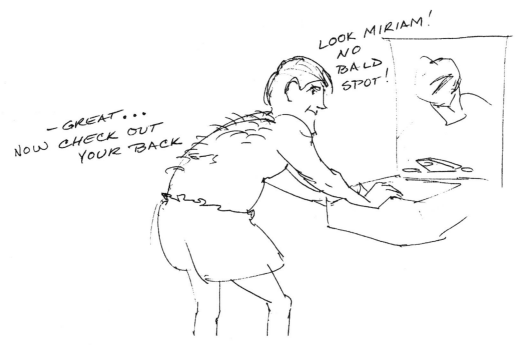

instead of freaking out about excess hair growth during pregnancy, men would welcome it—especially if they could get it to occur on their heads.

If Men Had Babies...

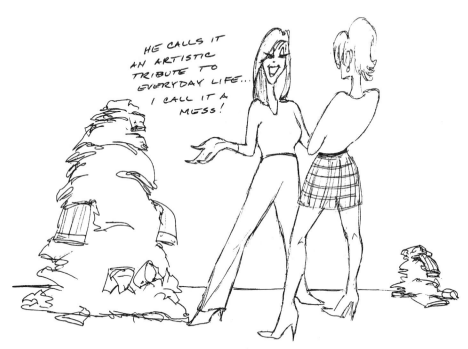

dressers would become obsolete. Men would just drop baby clothes on the kitchen floor, the den floor, the living room floor. . .wherever they changed the baby last.

If Men Had Babies...

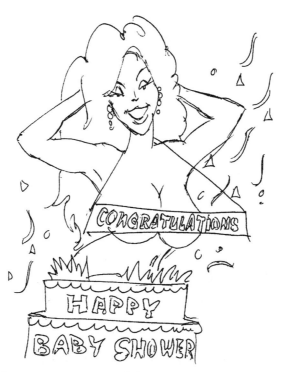

in lieu of baby shower favors, men would have a stripper popping out of a cake.

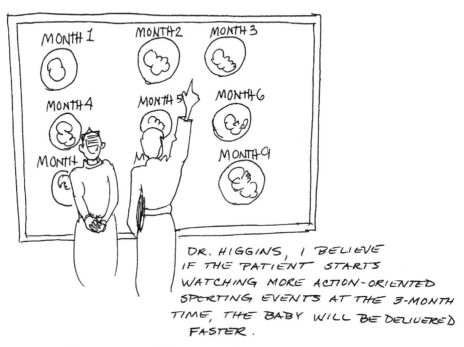

millions of dollars would be awarded to the scientist
who could shorten the length of pregnancy.

If Men Had Babies...

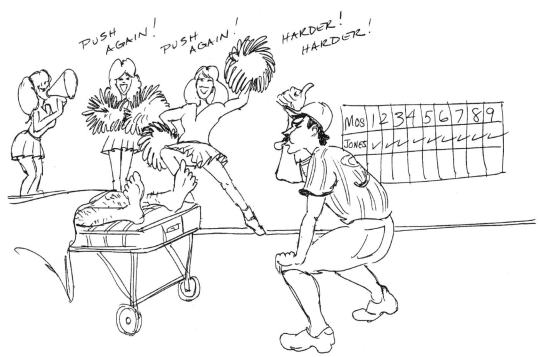

delivery rooms would have bleachers for the patient's buddies and cheerleaders.

If Men Had Babies...

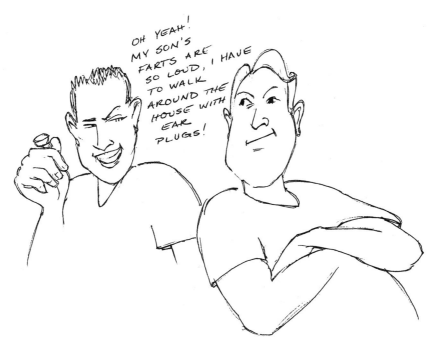

instead of bragging about baby's first step, first word and tooth, they'd brag about baby's first fart, burp, and spit.

If Men Had Babies...

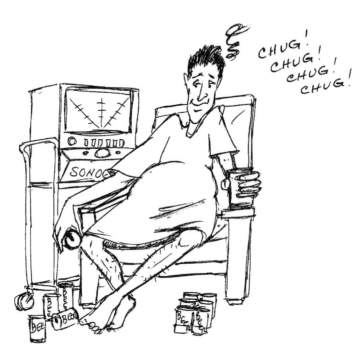

getting a sonogram would be like pledging a fraternity.
They'd be told to chug four mugs of beer and hold it in for an hour.

If Men Had Babies...

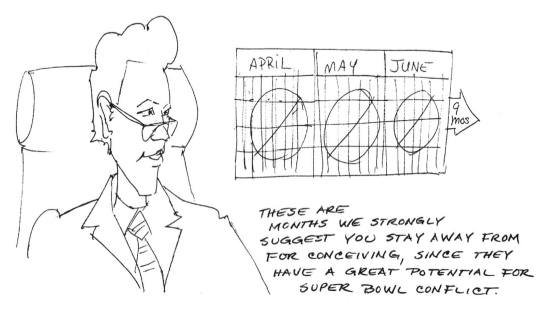

THESE ARE MONTHS WE STRONGLY SUGGEST YOU STAY AWAY FROM FOR CONCEIVING, SINCE THEY HAVE A GREAT POTENTIAL FOR SUPER BOWL CONFLICT.

all babies would be born in February.
(They couldn't be born in January because of the Super Bowl.
And don't forget college basketball tournaments in March,
opening day for baseball in April, NBA playoffs in May . . . you get the idea.)

If Men Had Babies...

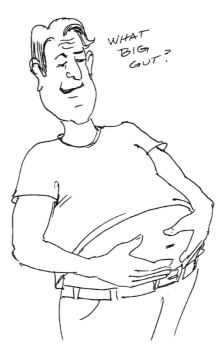

instead of being supportive of their friends during pregnancy, they'd say,
"Man, your gut is huge!"

If Men Had Babies...

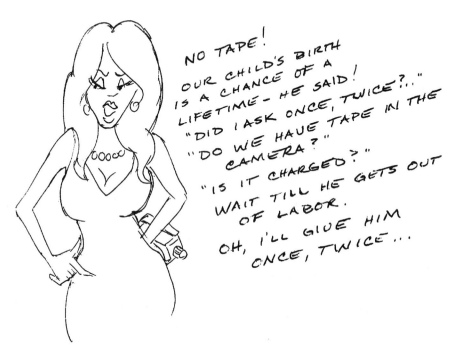

births would never get videotaped.
As usual, men would forget to load the tape.

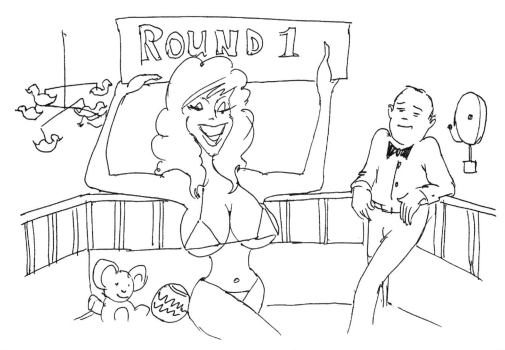

all playpens for twins would come equipped with a referee, a bell,
one black diaper and one white diaper, and two sets of mini boxing gloves.

If Men Had Babies...

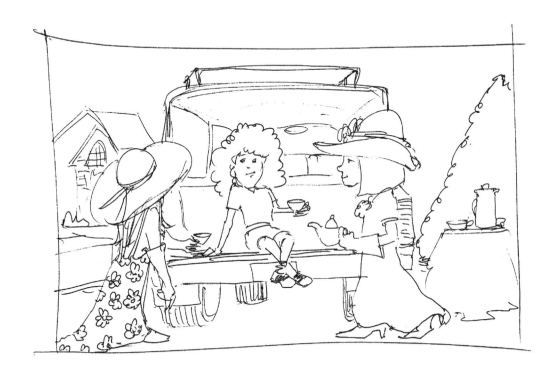

instead of tea parties, little girls would host tailgate parties.

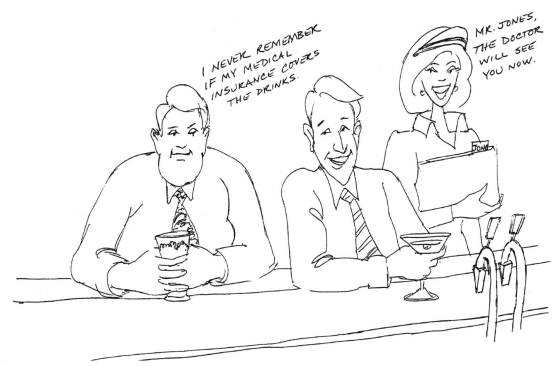

doctors' waiting rooms would have bar stools and serve hard liquor.

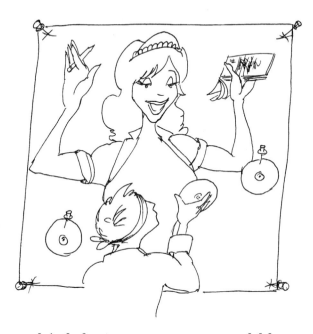

birthday party games would be:
- pin the hooters on the waitress   - musical remotes
- scissors, rock, karate chop   - hit the piñata with a 12-gauge

If Men Had Babies...

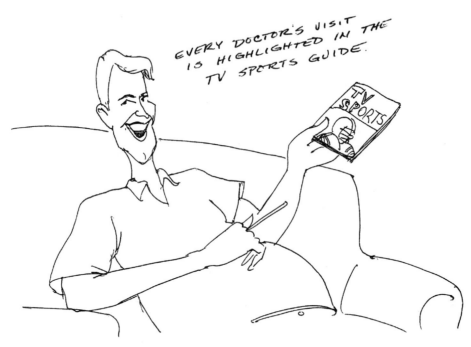

EVERY DOCTOR'S VISIT IS HIGHLIGHTED IN THE TV SPORTS GUIDE.

since men can't even remember their wives' birthdays, the only way they'd remember a doctor's appointment is if it coincided with a major sporting event.

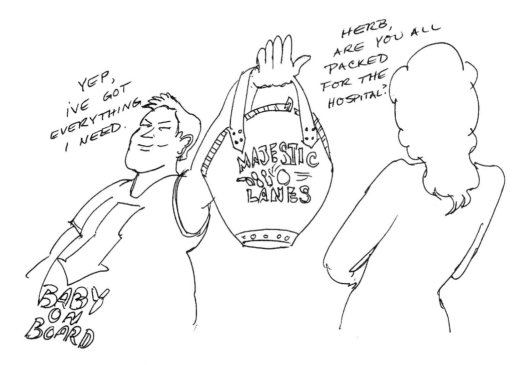

they would prepack an overnight bag *only* if there was a bowling alley at the hospital.

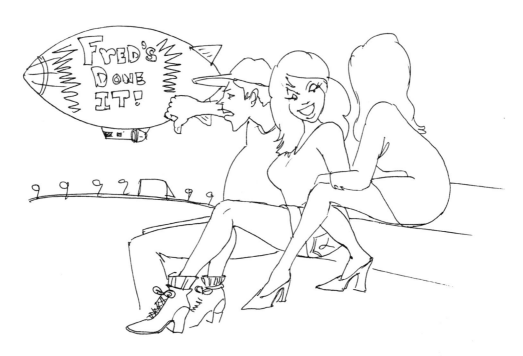

instead of mailing out formal birth announcements,
they'd announce their new arrivals on blimps.

If Men Had Babies...

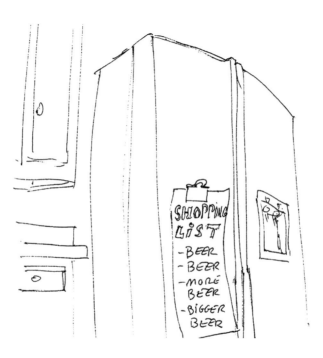

shopping lists for the family would look like this:
- beer   - pretzels   - more beer

If Men Had Babies...

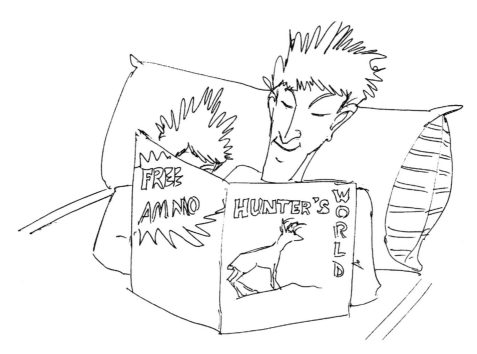

instead of Mother Goose bedtime stories,
they'd read articles from hunting magazines to their kids.

If Men Had Babies...

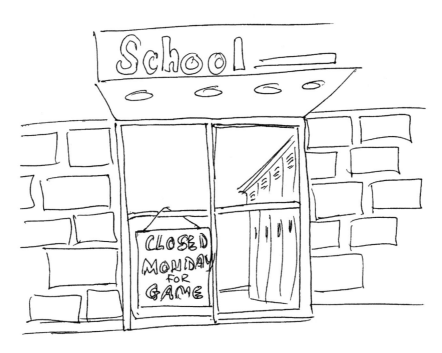

back-to-school night would never be scheduled on a Monday
from September to December (Monday Night Football!!!).

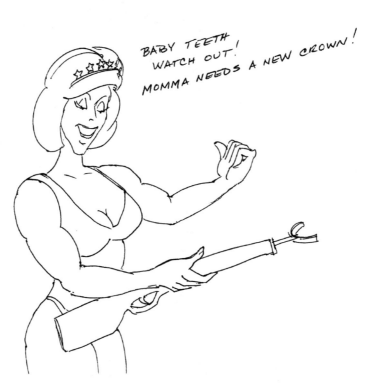

tooth fairies would be referred to as "tooth terminators."

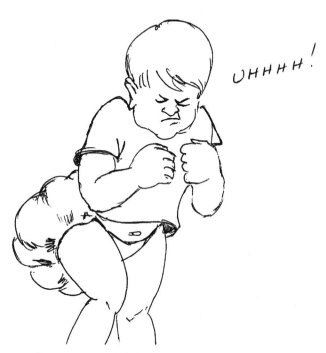

UHHHH!

diaper bags would be a thing of the past—
men would just order their kids to hold it in until they got home.

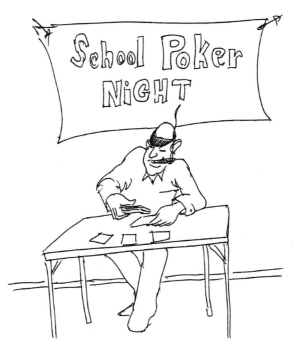

there would be no more bake sales.
Schools would have poker tables set up for fundraisers.

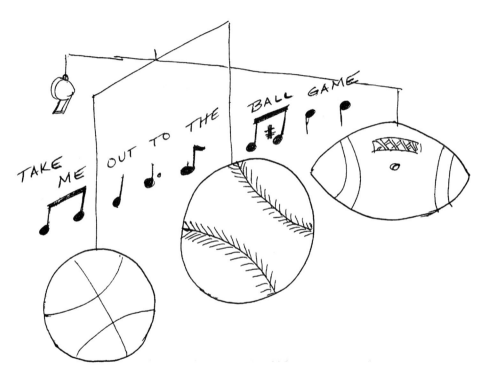

all musical baby mobiles would play "*Take Me Out to the Ball Game.*"

If Men Had Babies...

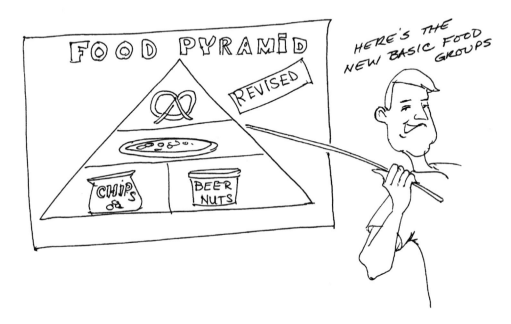

the four basic food groups would be:

♦ bread and cereal = pretzels ♦ milk products = pizza with extra cheese

♦ fruits and vegetables = potato chips ♦ protein = beer nuts

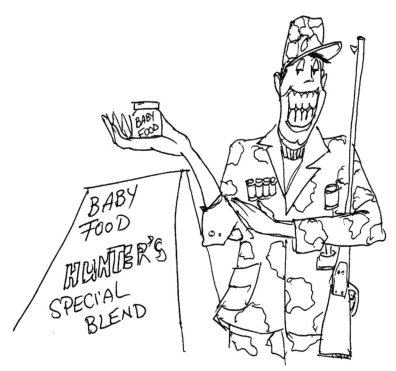

chicken and turkey baby food flavors would be replaced by buffalo and venison.

If Men Had Babies...

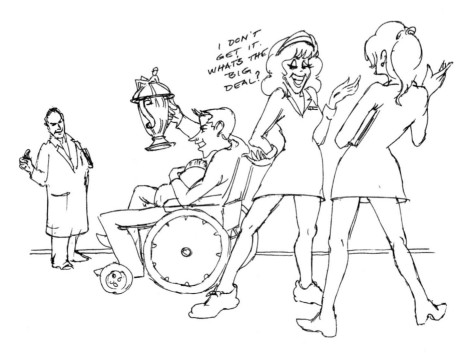

the free diaper bag hospitals give out with a new baby would be no more.
Men would expect a trophy, engraved: "for all of his hard work."

If Men Had Babies...

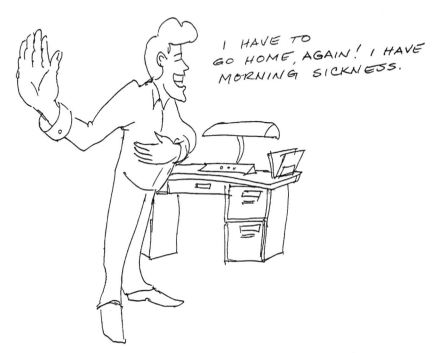

in accordance with a new law, "paternity leave"
would start in the first month of pregnancy.

If Men Had Babies...

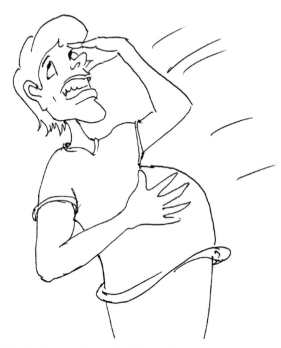

because of their low thresholds of pain, men wouldn't need epidurals. They'd pass out cold after the first contraction.

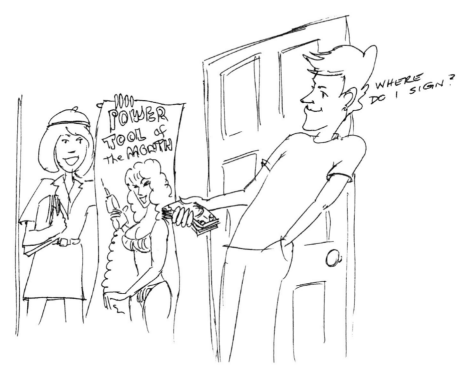

instead of selling cookies to raise money, little girls would sell power tools.

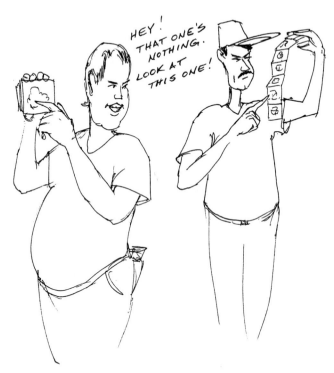

in addition to height and weight, baby boys' birth certificates would list penis size.

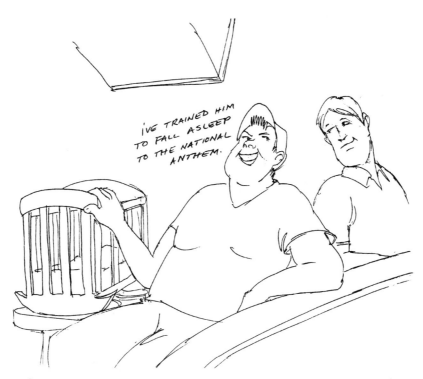

play groups would have to be held at sports bars.

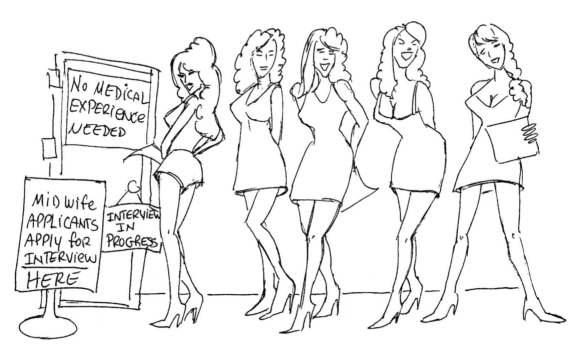

instead of interviewing midwives with their formal resumés,
men would download them naked on the Internet and then choose.

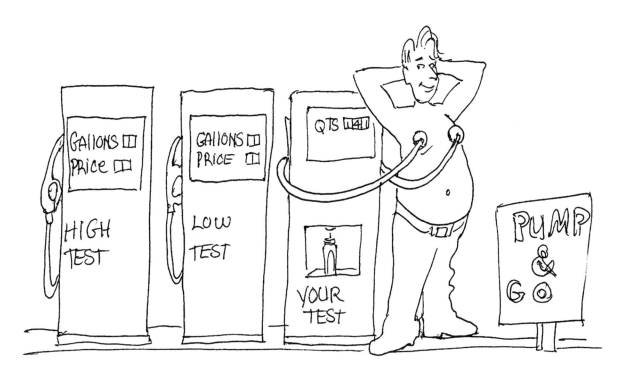

gas stations would come equipped with coin-operated breast pumps.

nursery rhymes would have a masculine slant...

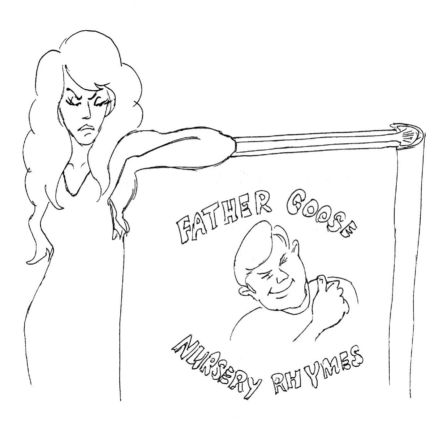

93

Big fat Jack Horner
sat in a corner
eating day-old pizza pie.
He sucked on his thumb
and thought of a dumb,
blond waitress he wanted to try.

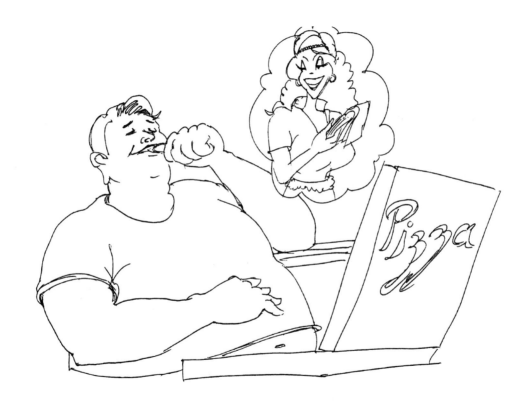

Jack and Bill
climbed up a hill
to lug two tons of water.
Jack fell down
and broke his crown.
And Bill said,
"Get the !@#* up and act like a man."

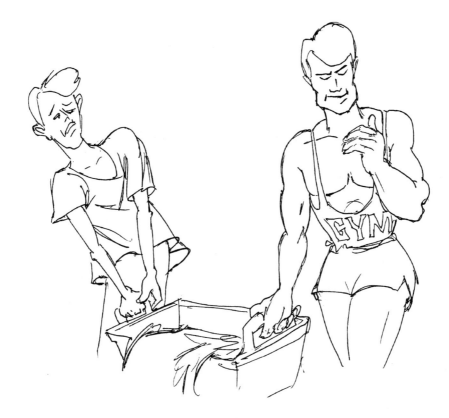

Little Miss Muffet
sat on a tuffet,
eating her curds and whey.
Along came a spider
that sat down beside her,
till her big brother took out his magnum
and blew him away!

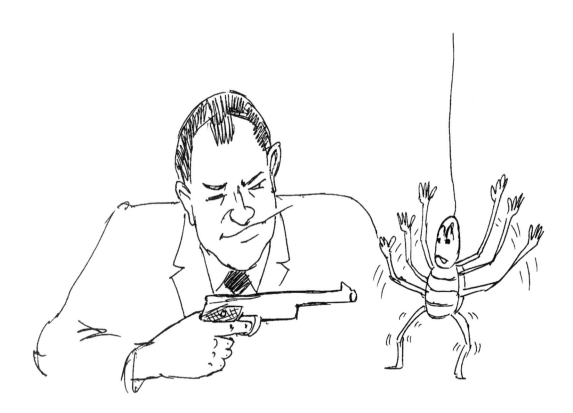

Three blind mice,
three blind mice.
See how they run,
see how they run.
They all ran after the farmer's wife,
her big brave husband grabbed a knife,
you've never seen so much blood in your life.
Three dead mice.

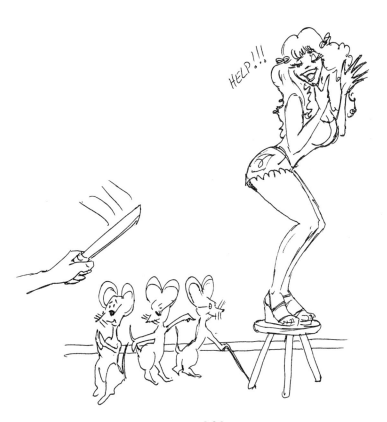

Mary had a big ole ram,
his fleece was black as coal.
And everywhere that Mary went. . .
''Bucky'' made sure no one
tried to mess with her.

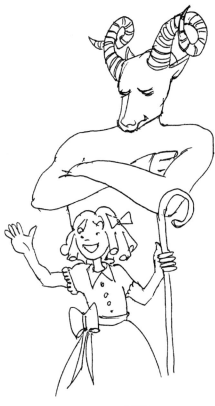

103

Humpty Dumpty sat on a wall.
Humpty Dumpty had a great fall.
All the king's horses
and all the king's men. . .
fried up some sausage and made an omelet.

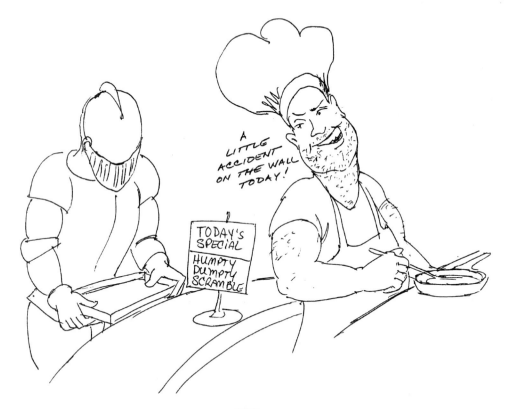

105

Rock-a-bye baby on the eighth hole,
when the ball rolls across the green knoll,
you'll stay asleep,
tucked in real tight,
while daddy plays golf
then boozes all night.

GOODNIGHT

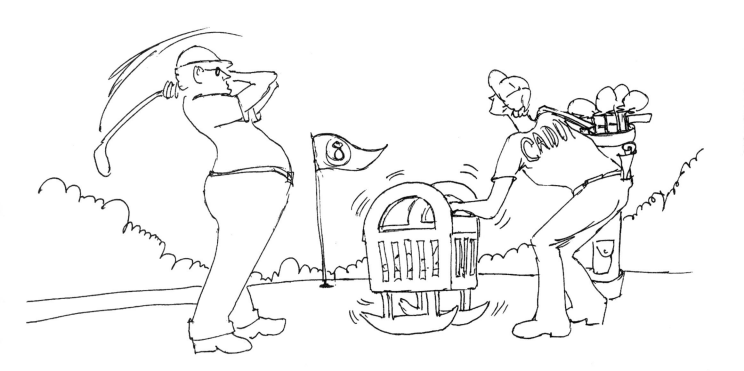

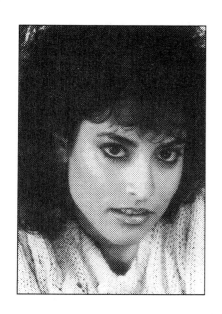

Karen Rostoker-Gruber is a published humorist. Her first book, "**The Unofficial College Survival Guide**," was published in 1992 by *Great Quotations*. Her second book, "**Remote Controls Are Better Than Women Because**," was published by *Longstreet Press* in 1993, and her third book, "**Telephones Are Better Than Men Because**," also published by *Longstreet Press*, came out in 1996. Karen has been a guest on the ***Ricki Lake Show*** and has promoted her books on radio shows coast to coast and in Canada.

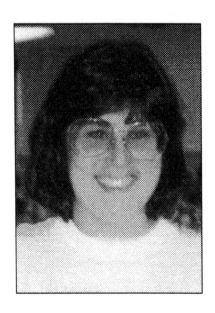

Gail Panzer-Salmanowitz has a master's degree in education. She specializes in science-oriented activities for children ages 7-12 and writes curriculum for the Board of Education in Elizabeth, New Jersey.

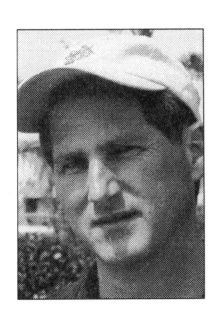

Jim Gallagher is a nationally recognized portrait artist/illustrator. He studied at the School of Visual Arts in New York with internationally-renowned illustrator Jack Potter. He considers his display at the Hard Rock Café to be one of his most significant accomplishments. He is a member of the Society of Illustrators.

TITLES BY CCC PUBLICATIONS

PARTY / CARTOON BOOKS - Retail $4.99 - $6.99

101 SIGNS/SPENDING TOO MUCH TIME W/ CAT
ARE WE DYSFUNCTIONAL YET?
ARE YOU A SPORTS NUT?
BETTER HALF, The
BOOK OF WHITE TRASH, The
BUT OSSIFER, IT'S NOT MY FAULT
CAT OWNER'S SHAPE-UP MANUAL
CYBERGEEK IS CHIC
DIFFERENCE BETWEEN MEN & WOMEN, The
FITNESS FANATICS
FLYING FUNNIES
GOLFAHOLICS
GOOD FOR NOTHIN' MEN
GO TO HEALTH!
IF MEN HAD BABIES...
LOVE & MARRIAGE & DIVORCE
LOVE DAT CAT
MALE BASHING: WOMEN'S FAVORITE PASTIME
MARITAL BLISS & OTHER OXYMORONS
MORE THINGS YOU CAN DO WITH A USELESS MAN
OFFICE FROM HELL, The
OH BABY!
PMS CRAZED: TOUCH ME AND I'LL KILL YOU!
SLICK EXCUSES FOR STUPID SCREW-UPS
SMART COMEBACKS FOR STUPID QUESTIONS
SO, YOU'RE GETTING MARRIED
SO, YOU'RE HAVING A BABY
TECHNOLOGY BYTES!
THINGS/DO WITH/USELESS MAN "G-Rated"
THINGS YOU'LL NEVER HEAR THEM SAY
WHY GOD MAKES BALD GUYS
WHY MEN ARE CLUELESS
YOUR COMPUTER THINKS YOU'RE AN IDIOT

GAG / BLANK BOOKS - Retail $4.99 - $5.99

ALL/WAYS MEN/SMARTER THAN WOMEN (blank)
ALL/WAYS WOMEN/SMARTER THAN MEN (blank)
COMPLETE GUIDE/RETIREMENT'S GREAT ACTIVITIES
COMPLETE GUIDE TO SEX AFTER 30 (blank)

COMPLETE GUIDE TO SEX AFTER 40 (blank)
COMPLETE GUIDE TO SEX AFTER 50 (blank)
COMPLETE GUIDE TO SEX AFTER BABY (blank)
COMPLETE GUIDE TO SEX AFTER MARRIAGE (blank)
COMPLETE GUIDE TO OVER-THE-HILL SEX (blank)
LAST DIET BOOK, The (gag)

AGE RELATED / OVER THE HILL - Retail $4.99 - $6.99

30 - DEAL WITH IT
40 - DEAL WITH IT
50 - DEAL WITH IT
60 - DEAL WITH IT
OVER THE HILL - DEAL WITH IT!
CRINKLED & WRINKLED
RETIREMENT: THE GET EVEN YEARS
SENIOR CITIZEN'S SURVIVAL GUIDE, The
WELCOME TO YOUR MIDLIFE CRISIS
YIKES, IT'S ANOTHER BIRTHDAY
YOU KNOW YOU'RE AN OLD FART WHEN...
YOUNGER MEN ARE BETTER THAN RETIN-A

MINI BOOKS (4 x 6) Retail $4.99 - $6.99

"?" [question mark book]
IT'S A MAD MAD MAD SPORTS WORLD
LITTLE BOOK OF CORPORATE LIES, The
LITTLE BOOK OF ROMANTIC LIES, The
LITTLE INSTRUCTION BOOK OF RICH & FAMOUS
NOT TONIGHT DEAR, I HAVE A COMPUTER
OLD, FAT, WHITE GUY'S GUIDE TO EBONICS, The
SINGLE WOMEN vs. MARRIED WOMEN
TAKE A WOMAN'S WORD FOR IT

TRADE PAPERBACKS Retail $4.99 - $7.99

50 WAYS TO HUSTLE YOUR FRIENDS
1001 WAYS TO PROCRASTINATE
ABSOLUTE LAST CHANCE DIET BOOK
BOTTOM HALF, The
EVERYTHING I KNOW/LEARNED/TRASH TALK TV
GETTING OLD SUCKS!

GETTING EVEN W/ ANSWERING MACH
GREATEST ANSWERING MACHINE MESSAGES
HOW TO ENTERTAIN PEOPLE YOU HATE
HOW TO GET FREE FOOD IN COLLEGE
HOW TO REALLY PARTY!
HOW TO SURVIVE A JEWISH MOTHER
HOW TO TALK/WAY OUT OF/TRAFFIC TICKET
IT'S BETTER/OVER THE HILL THAN UNDER IT
I WISH I DIDN'T...
KILLER BRAS
LADIES, START YOUR ENGINES
LIFE'S MOST EMBARRASSING MOMENTS
HORMONES FROM HELL
HORMONES FROM HELL II
HUSBANDS FROM HELL
MEN LOVE FOOTBALL/WOMEN LOVE FOREPLAY
NEVER A DULL CARD
PEOPLE WATCHER'S FIELD GUIDE
RED HOT MONOGAMY
SHARING THE ROAD WITH IDIOTS
UGLY TRUTH ABOUT MEN
UNOFFICIAL WOMEN'S DIVORCE GUIDE
WHAT DO WE DO NOW?? (New Parents)
WHY MEN DON'T HAVE A CLUE
WORK SUCKS!

"ON THE EDGE" - Retail $4.99 - $6.99

ART OF MOONING, The
COMPLETE BOOGER BOOK, The
COMPLETE WIMP'S GUIDE TO SEX, The
FARTING
SEX AND YOUR STARS
SEX IS A GAME
SEXY CROSSWORD PUZZLES
SIGNS YOUR SEX LIFE IS DEAD
THE TOILET ZONE
THINGS/DO WITH/USELESS MAN "R-Rated"
TOTAL BASTARD'S GUIDE TO GOLF, The
YOU KNOW HE'S/WOMANIZING SLIMEBALL WHEN...